Love Your Diet

Vitamins & Minerals

K.J.R. Alexander

Contents

Introduction

Vitamins and Minerals is a supplement to the Love Your Diet books. The purpose is to give dieters an optional quick reference to vitamins and minerals to better understand why some foods are nutritious and others are not. Today's consumer needs more information to make informed decisions while the basics of nutrition are not readily available. The Love Your Diet program emphasizes how essential balanced nutrition is to excess fat loss, weight maintenance, and to health in general. The big picture of nutrition proves how extreme diets, excessive fast food, and too much starch and sugar deprive the body of needed nutrients. The potential starch and sugar addict in everyone cannot argue with vitamins and minerals.

It is often said that all animals readily go for sugar except cats. Cats are naturally finicky eaters, preferring live mice and cream. And we can observe many animals such as honey bees and humming birds feeding on sweet nectar. While the statement is too generalized, it does capture the powerful and primal attraction to sugar and starch in carbohydrates. More on starch and sugar addiction and the effects on food choices are explained in Love Your Diet's *Light Fantastic* and *Calories & Real Foods*.

The information here is condensed into easy to scan tables, which include introductions to the vitamin or mineral, its function, samples of foods with the nutrient, symptoms of deficiency, and recommended daily intake. Deficiencies are interesting because they indicate how science identified the function of the vitamin or mineral when missing; they also provide additional information showing how hard the nutrient works in the body when it is adequate. Scan the tables and keep them handy for future reference in reading food labels or planning menus. Today's dieter needs such basic information in order to make healthy choices and to be able to follow the continual changes in the science of foods.

After the vitamin and mineral charts, two tables are included. Both include explanatory notes at the end of the table. The first one, *Recommended Daily Allowances & Adequate Intakes for Nutrients*, summarizes daily needs for the average adult, along with known toxicities of supplementation. The other one, *Nutrition Power*, compares enriched white flour with wheat germ, wheat germ oil, and wheat bran, the nutrients removed in refining. Also included are dairy foods, liver, and brewers yeast. Adding these foods to the diet boosts nutrition power. The less familiar ones are briefly discussed below.

Wheat Germ, the center of a grain of wheat, contains nutrients removed from refined white flour. Raw or toasted, a little sprinkled on cereal, added to juice, or added to baking products can help boost nutrition. The oil from the seed, wheat germ oil, at 20 mg per tablespoon, is the richest known natural source of Vitamin E. A teaspoon of wheat germ oil every day or so therefore increases Vitamin E. Importantly, it illustrates the need to eat whole wheat and other whole grain nutrients.

Wheat Bran, the outer covering of a grain of wheat is one of the richest sources of high fiber. A tablespoon in a glass of juice or on cereal adds additional fiber and nutrition to the day.

Brewers Yeast, an unleavening or nonrising yeast used in the brewing process, is included in the *Nutrition Power* table because it is commonly recommended by nutritionists as a supplement for its rich supply of 17 vitamins, 14 minerals, and 16 amino acids as well as RNA, ribonucleic acid, a substance that gives cell direction or "informs" the cell what to do. Brewers yeast comes in flaked, powdered, or tablet form. There are also nutritional food yeasts which may have a milder taste. Some also have added B12 cobalamin to round out the B vitamin complex. Just one or two tablespoons a day can enrich daily metabolism. Since the yeast is high in phosphorous and phosphorous needs to be balanced with calcium, a calcium food should also be used along with the yeast.

Also helpful to understanding the importance of a balanced diet is to take a quick look at some of the current terms in the science of nutrition such as antioxidants, carotenoids, polyphenols, and phytoestrogens.

Free Radicals and Antioxidants

Free radicals have been identified as substances potentially harmful to the body. They can damage DNA and RNA, which direct cell actions. By obstructing proper cell repair and replacement, they can also cause disease and are seen as the cause of many health problems.

Free radicals are chemicals produced by body metabolism in reaction to harmful substances. They are created by the process of oxidation and are also known as oxidants. The oxidant, or free radical, is minus one electron and is therefore unstable, grabbing an electron from a stable molecule, which then in turn is unstable and needs an electron which it gains from yet another molecule and so on, causing a chain reaction. The body naturally creates some free radicals as part of the immune system to attack invading viruses and bacteria. However, many conditions and substances in the environment also trigger free radical attacks, which are harmful to healthy cells. These include, for example, pollutants, toxic chemicals, radiation, pesticides, drugs, and cleaning agents. Stress and sudden high intensity exercise also create free radicals.

Free radicals are stopped by the body with substances called antioxidants, which stop or prevent the oxidation process creating free radicals. Antioxidants stop the damage of free radical chain reactions by being able to give up an electron without becoming unstable, without needing another electron. They consume free radicals, stopping the process of chain reactions. Powerful antioxidants are Vitamins C, E and beta carotene. The mineral selenium is another primary antioxidant necessary to the function of antioxidant enzyme systems. Other antioxidants in fruits and vegetables are phytochemicals, polyphenals, and phytoestrogens.

Vitamin C or ascorbic acid is a water soluble vitamin in citrus fruits such as oranges, limes, lemons, and grapefruit. Other sources include spinach, broccoli, cabbage, and strawberries. Some of the many benefits of Vitamin C are described in the vitamin chart.

Vitamin E or d-alpha tocopherol, is a fat soluble vitamin also described more in the vitamin chart. Some sources include nuts and seeds, whole grains, apricots, and vegetable oils. The alpha tocopherol form of Vitamin E is considered to be the most effective nutritionally.

The many different **carotenoids**, such as beta carotene, from which the body manufactures Vitamin A are major antioxidants. Carotenoids are obtained from dark orange and green fruits and vegetables such as apricots, sweet potatoes, and spinach. Vitamin A is also found in animal products in a preformed state (the animals have already changed carotenoids to Vitamin A) such as in meats, eggs, cream, and butter (cream and butter have both carotenoids and preformed Vitamin A). *The difference is that preformed Vitamin A is not an antioxidant. The carotenoids and beta carotene are the antioxidants.*

Although not a direct antioxidant, the preformed Vitamin A in the human body works with Vitamin E. Vitamin A is produced in the upper intestine and stored in the liver as an oil soluble vitamin. Fish liver oil contains very rich amounts of preformed Vitamin A as well as omega 3 fatty acids.

The best sources of these antioxidants are from natural foods and moderate levels in vitamin supplements. *High megadoses* in supplements may actually do the opposite and increase free radical action and are therefore not recommended.

Phytochemicals are substances in fruits and vegetables that protect them from too much sun. In the body, they are thought to help block processes that lead to various cancers. Tomatoes have an estimated 10,000 phytochemicals. Other sources are fruits and vegetables such as strawberries, grapes, raspberries, brussels sprouts, broccoli, and cauliflower.

Polyphenols are another group of antioxidants thought to help protect against heart disease and stomach and lung cancers. Sources include onions, yams, strawberries, apples, wine, coffee, and black and green teas.

Phytoestrogens are a weak estrogen substance in plants that have been thought to help protect against hormonal cancers such as breast and prostate cancer. Phytoestrogens are found, as well as in other plants, in soybeans and soybean products such as soy milk, tofu, and soy sauce. Such soybean "estrogen" has also been used to successfully treat symptoms of menopause and PMS or premenstrual syndrome. However, it is now thought that estrogen based breast cancer may be exacerbated by plant estrogens so that high concentrations should be avoided by breast cancer patients. Research continues.

The increasing free radical factors in the environment increase the need for fresh foods that provide antioxidants that stop and block free radical damage. On the Love Your Diet program, let your body lead you to the bright colors of the many fruits and vegetables in the produce section. The more intense the color, the more antioxidants they provide; deep purple, bright orange, and dark green are rich in antioxidants.

The following vitamin and mineral charts are designed for conceptual or intuitive insight into the molecular world of nutrition and metabolism as well as to provide a quick reference. They will help in understanding why Love Your Diet works so well and provides the foundation to maintain lifelong nutrition and weight control.

VITAMINS & MINERALS

VITAMINS

Terms

RDA   Recommended Daily Allowance - standardized amount for daily intake preventing deficiency.
AI   Adequate Intake – standardized amount for daily intake preventing deficiency.
IU   International Unit – standardized amount
Supplement Supplementary to diet: taken in pills or other form. Amount safely taken to increase intake.
Toxicity   Amount which is toxic.

Vitamin A

Description	What It Does	Sample Food Sources	Deficiency Effects
Yellow fat-soluble substance found in carotene, which is converted to Vitamin A during digestion. Vitamin A is of two types: that which is not yet formed but is still carotene (provitamin A) and that which is already formed in animal products (preformed Vitamin A). Carotenes are powerful antioxidants.	Maintains skin and surface of all mucous membranes. Forms visual purple in eye for night vision. Fights infections and disease, speeds wound healing. Facilitates cell development and RNA production.	Leafy green and yellow vegetables and deeply colored fruits. Dairy products. Liver, fish liver oil. Carrots, corn, asparagus, broccoli, dandelion greens, kale, hot chili pepper, paprika, spinach, sweet potato, pumpkin, squash, tomatoes, apricots, cherries, mangos, papayas, peaches. Egg yolk, cheese, butter, milk, crab, halibut, mackerel, salmon, oysters.	Night blindness, dry skin, eye infections, skin blemishes, increased risk of infection and disease.

RDA/AI: 5000 IU & 700-900 RE (Retinol Equivalent) Preformed or already formed Vitamin A also expressed in RE or Retinol Equivalents. One RE comparable to about five IUs.

Toxicity: None for natural carotenes and natural foods.
Preformed Vitamin A toxic in large doses over long periods of time (100,000 IU).
Pregnant women limit preformed Vitamin A to 5,000 IU.

Vitamin B Complex

Description	What They Do	Sample Food Sources	Deficiency Effects
There are eight B-Complex Vitamins: B1-Thiamine B2-Riboflavin B3-Niacin B5- Pantothenic Acid* B6-Pyridoxine B12-Cobalamin Biotin* Folate* Not one of B-Complex Vitamins but working closely with them: Choline* Inositol* PABA* Para-aminobenzoic Acid.	The B-Complex Vitamins are synergistic coenzymes enabling many metabolic processes. They help maintain the nervous system and prevent mental and nervous disorders, produce red blood cells, maintain immunity and act as antioxidants, regulate cardiovascular functions, supply muscles with energy, synthesize nucleic acid and DNA, maintain skin, hair, and liver.	Food sources are liver and organ meats, brewers yeast, meat, poultry, seafood, beans, nuts, seeds, whole grains, eggs, yogurt, milk products, fruits, vegetables.	Nervousness, irritability, depression, dementia. Nerve disorders and brain damage. Nerve inflammation and pain. Graying, thinning hair. Dry flaky skin and skin blemishes. Insomnia, anemia, high cholesterol, weakness, fatigue, kidney failure, cardiac failure, reduced immunity to infections and disease.

* Available in foods and manufactured in body

The B-Complex Vitamins are grouped together because they occur in foods together and function together. *They are synergistic; each works with all the others to be effective.* B-vitamin intake in natural foods contains the proper balance in providing complete B-complex. An increase in only one B-vitamin, as in supplements, can deplete the others or be ineffective because the others are missing. *Therefore, any individual B-vitamin taken in pills or capsules should also be accompanied by all of the other B-vitamins in a B-complex supplement to prevent deficiencies in other B-vitamins.* They are water soluble and not stored by the body so a daily supply is needed from food or supplements. Sugar and alcohol deplete B-vitamins increasing need. Though some B-vitamins are produced by the body, this production is dependent on dietary B-vitamins.

B1 Thiamine

Description	What it Does	Sample Food Sources	Deficiency Effects
thy eh men **thy** eh mean White, water soluble, crystalline compound.	Works with enzymes (coenzyme) to metabolize carbohydrates and amino acids. Maintains nerves and nervous system and helps mental attitude. Helps maintain red blood cells, convert glucose into energy, maintain smooth and skeletal muscles. Helps detoxify lead, repels insects and fleas. Stabilizes appetite.	Milk, yogurt, grain seed coats, whole grains, enriched flour, peas, cauliflower, liver, meat, poultry, lobster, salmon, cheese, eggs, peanuts, fruits and berries, pinto beans, black beans, soy beans, brewers yeast.	Irritability, mood swing, mental confusion, anorexia, heart irregularity, disturbed vision, staggering walk, numbness in feet and legs, low blood pressure. Causes beriberi disease involving pain and swelling in extremities, emaciation, body swelling, nerve disorders. Extreme: kidney failure, heart failure.

RDA/AI: 1.2 -1.2 mg.   Supplement: 1.5 – 10 mg.
Toxicity of large doses: None known.

B2 Riboflavin

Description

Rye bow flay vin

Orange-yellow, water soluble, crystalline compound

B2-riboflavin is destroyed by sunlight but survives cooking and is not naturally abundant in foods but often added in enriched products.

Exercise increases need.

What It Does

Antioxidant and coenzyme. Protects against free radicals. Helps regulate cell respiration and metabolism. Aids iron absorption and protects against anemia. Known as the exercise vitamin, it is depleted with intense exercise, increasing need. Helps maintain skin, hair, eyes.

Sample Food Sources

Milk, yogurt, cottage cheese, liver, organ meats, brewers yeast. Whole grains, enriched flour. Small amounts in leafy vegetables, almonds, filberts, eggs, fresh salmon and mackerel, fruits, meat, chocolate, beer*, wine*.

Deficiency Effects

Red, burning tongue, cracks in corners of mouth, burning eyes, eye fatigue, sensitivity to light. Face and genital eczema. Dizziness, trembling, digestive disturbance, lack of vitality, oily skin, depression and weight loss, inability to urinate. Slow growth. Also results in pellagra, which is also a disease in niacin deficiency (see under niacin). Deficiency common in elderly, alcoholics, those on lasix, antacids, psychotropics or tranquilizers, those consuming bisulfite preservatives in meat and wine, and hypothyroidism.

RDA/AI: 1.1 – 1.3 mg.   Supplement: up to 20 - 100 mg.   Exercisers: 2 – 2. 5 mg.
Toxicity in high doses: None known.

*Beer and wine in the lists are for interest and not intended to indicate using as a source of vitamins.

B3 Niacin

Description	What It Does	Food Sources	Deficiency Effects
Nye eh sin	Coenzyme to energy metabolism. Helps maintain nervous system, circulation, and digestive tissues. Vasodilator. Nicotinic acid only: lowers cholesterol and blood pressure, detoxifies pollutants, alcohol, narcotics. Helps in schizophrenia and mental disorders, protects against recurring heart attacks, benefits diabetes and arthritis. Skin maintenance and repair. Aids production of sex hormones. Produced by body from amino acid tryptophan (60 mg. yields one mg. niacin.)	Foods: Liver, brewers yeast, wheat bran, whole grains, enriched flour, bulgur, rice, wild rice, peanuts, lentils, potatoes, eggs, meat, poultry, crab, oysters, shrimp, halibut, salmon, mackerel. Smaller amounts in milk products, fruits, and vegetables: apricots, dates, corn, cauliflower, broccoli, mushrooms, peas, squash, tomatoes, sesame seeds, beer, wine.	Deficiency: Fatigue and muscle weakness, indigestion, appetite loss, skin blemishes, canker sores, insomnia, irritability, headaches, tender gums, depression. Severe deficiency results in pellagra: exhibited by nervous disorder and dementia, dermatitis, nerve dysfunction, tremors, diarrhea. Excessive starch and sugar intake depletes niacin.
Nicotinic Acid Nicotinamide Niacinamide Clear, water soluble, crystalline compound			

RDA/AI: 14 - 16 mg.   Supplement: 20 - 100 mg
Toxicity of large doses: Temporary "niacin flush" in reddening of skin in face, neck, arms, and chest with 100 mg. or more. Large doses over period of time may cause liver malfunction, glucose intolerance. Medical supervision required for large doses of a maximum of 2 grams.

B5 Pantothenic Acid

Description	What It Does	Food Sources	Deficiency Effects
pan teh **thin** ick Pantethine Pantothenic acid Oily hydroxy acid (properties of both alcohol and acid). In foods and manufactured in body.	Coenzyme in fatty acid metabolism. Metabolism of adrenal hormones and cellular energy. Lowers cholesterol and triglycerides (pantothine) and protects against cardiovascular disease, inhibits blood clots and irregular heartbeat. Helps prevent hair loss and graying of hair. Slows aging and wrinkles. Speeds wound healing. Boosts athletic energy. Essential in formation of cholesterol and fatty acids. Anti-stress. Alcohol detoxifier. Synthesized in intestines by bacteria. Highest concentrations in brain.	Liver, brewers yeast, yogurt, wheat germ, whole wheat, bran, rice, oats, poultry, meat, crab, oysters, halibut, mackerel, salmon, oysters, fruits, berries, nuts, sunflower seeds, beans, vegetables, mushrooms, broccoli, eggs, milk and milk products, beer, wine.	Rare because abundant. May occur when intestines lack intestinal bacteria needed to synthesize. Insomnia, depression, fatigue, motor disturbances, reduced immunity.

RDA/AI: 5 mg.   Supplement: 10 – 100 mg.   Toxicity: None known.

B6 Pyridoxine

Description	What It Does	Food Sources	Deficiency Effects
pier eh **dock** *seen* Pyridoxine Pyridoxal Pyridoxamine Consists of three water soluble compounds (above)	Essential coenzyme to over 60 enzymes. Super coenzyme and immune booster. Needed for RNA, DNA, protein, and immune cell synthesis. Needed for absorption of Vitamin B12-cobalamin and production of red blood cells. Helps maintain brain neurotransmitters and nervous system, helps schizophrenia. Anti-Convulsive. Helps PMS, birth-control users, morning sickness. Diuretic. Helps release glycogen from liver and muscles for energy. May be anticancer and helps control diabetes. Effective carpel tunnel treatment. Helps maintain nerve and muscle-skeletal functions.	Foods: Liver, brewers yeast, yogurt, wheat germ, whole wheat, bran, rice, oats, poultry, meat, crab, oysters, halibut, mackerel, salmon, fruits, berries, nuts, sunflower seeds, beans, mushrooms, broccoli, eggs, milk and milk products, beer, wine. Fortified cereals and fortified soy-based meat substitutes.	Nervousness, brain dysfunction. Anemia, low blood sugar and insulin sensitivity, irritability, depression, muscle weakness, numbness and cramps or temporary paralysis in limbs, cracks around mouth, dermatitis, hair loss, eye disturbances, water retention.

RDA/AI: 1.3 – 1.7 mg.   Supplement: 2 – 100 mg.

Toxicity: Toxic in large doses (2 grams) taken over prolonged periods. No megadoses. Reduces effect of levodopa given for Parkinson's disease.

B12 Cyanocobalamin

Description	What It Does	Food Sources	Deficiency Effects
Sy eh no co *bal* eh men Cobalamin Cyanocobalamin Deep red water-soluble solid. Only vitamin containing mineral element (cobalt). Cannot be produced synthetically. Cultured in molds or bacteria.	Coenzyme in nucleic acid metabolism. Aids conversion of carotene to Vitamin A. Works with folic acid in choline synthesis. Maintains nerve tissue. Alleviates neuropsychiatric disorders, prevents mental deterioration, fights viral and bacterial infections, anticancer esp. smoking-related, blocks adverse reactions of sulfites. Works with amino acids, Vitamin C, and pantothenic acid. Facilitates iron in producing red blood cells.	Liver and organ meats, yogurt, meat, poultry, eggs, milk, cottage cheese, fish, oysters, crab, salmon, mackerel. Fortified cereal.	Nerve disorders in reflex and coordination. Difficulty speaking and walking, soreness in arms and legs, nervousness, mood disorder, brain damage and psychosis. Anemia.

RDA/AI: 2.4 mcg.   Supplement: 5 – 50 mcg.   Toxicity: None known to 450 mg.

Folate

Description	What It Does	Food Sources	Deficiency Effects
foe late	Helps produce and maintain new cells. Synthesizes DNA and RNA in cells. Prevents changes to DNA. Anticancer. Prevents birth defects. Produces protein, which carries iron and helps form red blood cells. Works with Vitamins B12 and C in metabolism of proteins. Synthesized in intestine by bacteria.	Liver, brewers yeast, spinach, peas, yogurt, egg, cottage cheese, garbanzo beans, pinto beans, navy beans, lentils, black beans, peanuts, orange juice, whole grains, enriched cereals and grains, broccoli, cauliflower, cabbage.	Metabolic and digestive disorders, weakness, fatigue, graying hair, swollen tongue, anemia, birth defects, slow growth, high number of red blood cells. Smokers, elderly, deficient. Drugs such as anticonvulsants, sulfa drugs, oral contraceptives deplete.
Folic Acid Folacin Part of compounds of folates (foliage) in leafy green vegetables and higher plants. *Folate* is the naturally occurring B-vitamin in foods. *Folic Acid* is the synthetic form in supplements and fortified foods. In foods and manufactured in body.			

RDA/AI: 400 mcg.   Supplement: 400 - 1000 mcg.   Toxicity: None. If B12-cobalamin deficient, may cause neurological damage.

PABA — Para-Aminobenzoic Acid

Description	What It Does	Food Sources	Deficiency Effects
pair eh - eh me no ben *zoe* ick acid	Functions as a coenzyme in metabolism of proteins and in formation of red blood cells. Activates intestinal bacteria to produce folic acid. Folic acid then produces pantothenic acid. Also used as sunscreen in lotions and cosmetics.	Liver and organ meats, brewers yeast, wheat germ, molasses, yogurt, green leafy vegetables.	Digestive difficulty, irritability, fatigue, depression, nervousness, graying hair, headache, constipation. Sulfa drugs deplete intestinal bacteria and PABA.
Occurs in combination with folic acid. In foods and manufactured in body.			

RDA/AI: None.   Supplement: up to 30 mg.   Toxicity: None known but no high doses.

Choline

Description	What It Does	Food Sources	Deficiency Effects
koe *lean*	Important in fat metabolism and cholesterol functions. Maintains nerve sheaths and promotes nerve transmission. Helps regulate liver and gallbladder. Helps prevent hardening of the arteries.	Liver and organ meats, brewers yeast, wheat germ, eggs, spinach, cabbage, green beans, asparagus, white potato, sweet potato, whole wheat, rolled oats, meat.	High blood pressure, fatty deposits in liver, blockage of tubes of kidneys, artherosclerosis or hardening of the arteries.
Component of lecithin along with inositol. Lecithin manufactured in liver.			
In foods and manufactured in body			

RDA/AI: 550 mg.   Supplement: up to 3500 mg.   Toxicity: May deplete B6-pyridoxine and cause liver toxicity.

Inositol

Description	What It Does	Food Sources	Deficiency Effects
eh **no** *seh tall*	Works with choline to prevent hardening of the arteries and reduce blood cholesterol. Component of cell walls and cell function. Necessary for hair growth. Helps nourish brain cells, spinal cord nerve. Anti-anxiety.	Wheat germ, whole grains, brewers yeast, chicken, beans, nuts, oysters, grapefruit, oranges, cantaloupe, watermelon, strawberries, cabbage, cauliflower, spinach, lettuce, potato, sweet potato, liver, milk, eggs, halibut, salmon.	High blood cholesterol and hardening of the arteries, hair loss, eczema, eye problems.
White, sweet, crystalline solid. Found in many plants and seeds and in animal tissue.			
Component of lecithin along with choline.			
Prevalent in body.			
In foods and manufactured in body.			

RDA/AI: 500 – 1000 mg.   Supplement: up to 1000 mg.   Toxicity: None known.

Biotin

Description	What It Does	Food Sources	Deficiency Effects
bye eh tin Crystalline substance widely found in plant and animal tissue. In foods and manufactured in body.	Helps produce fatty acids and nucleic acid. Supports B12, folic acid, and pantothenic acid functions. Synthesized in intestines by bacteria.	Liver and organ meats, brewers yeast, eggs, rice, roquefort cheese, milk, bacon, ham, veal, crab, halibut, sardines, avocado, cantaloupe, grapes, oranges, peaches, strawberries, watermelon, peanuts, asparagus, green beans, carrots, raw cauliflower, red cabbage, mushrooms	Deficiency can be caused by eating large amounts of raw egg whites that bind with biotin (cooked eggs do not). Long term antibiotics deplete. Dermatitis, raised cholesterol, gray skin, insomnia, muscle pain, depression, loss of appetite.

RDA/AI: 30 mcg.   Supplement: 100 – 300 mcg.   Toxicity: None known.

Vitamin C

Description	What It Does	Food Sources	Deficiency Effects
Ascorbic acid. White, crystalline, water soluble.	Antioxidant. Increases immunity, anticancer, reduces effects of colds. Blocks nitrosamine formation in body (in cured meats, malt beverages, cosmetics). Prevents gum disease. Enhances antipsychotic drugs and controls oxidation of medicines. Helps mental disorders such as bipolar. Regulates water and electrolyte metabolism. Manufactures collagen, speeds wound healing. Asthma aid. Vital for metabolism, strengthens blood vessels, increase resistance to infections.	Citrus fruits, vegetables. Rosehips, oranges, grapefruit, lemon, lime, strawberries, black currants, guava, green pepper, red pepper, broccoli, brussels sprouts, asparagus, cauliflower, sweet potato, artichoke, tomato	Discovered when sailors in past centuries developed scurvy on long voyages due to lack of citrus fruits and Vitamin C. Eating limes prevented the problem. Scurvy symptoms are swollen and bleeding gums, extreme fatigue and listlessness, bruises and spots on the skin. Deficiency also causes nosebleeds, slow healing wounds, painful joints, wasting of muscles. 75% cancer patients deficient in Vitamin C.

RDA/AI: 60 - 90 mg. Supplement: 250 – 1,000 mg. (Take half-amounts twice daily for better absorption.

Toxicity: May cause diarrhea, abdominal pain, skin rash. Megadoses, such as 10,000 mg. daily over period of time, suddenly stopped, cause scurvy symptoms

Vitamin D

Description

Vitamin D is produced in the body by photosynthesis during the body's exposure to sunlight. The sun's ultraviolet rays change skin cholesterol to Vitamin D.

Also produced synthetically. Includes D1, D2, D3, etc. Fat soluble.

What It Does

Essential to calcium and phosphorous concentrations in the body enabling growth and maintenance of strong healthy bones. Necessary for children's proper bone growth. Contributes to functions of calcium and phosphorous in maintaining bones, nervous system, heart rhythm, and blood clotting. Cancer prevention and treatment. Helps immunity, psoriasis, elderly osteoporosis

Food Sources

Sources include sunshine, irradiated milk, egg yolks, liver, and fish liver oils.

Deficiency Effects

Causes rickets, disease in growing children where softening of bones, due to Vitamin D and calcium deficiency, causes bone deformity. Milk fortified with Vitamin D prevents this problem. At risk for deficiency: elderly, non-milk drinkers, lack of sun. Drugs depleting: anticonvulsant, cholesterol control, phenobarbital.

RDA: 400 IU   Supplement: 400 – 1,000 IU
Toxicity: Toxic in high doses. Nausea, vomiting, increased urination, diarrhea, drowsiness, calcification of heart, blood vessels, lungs. High blood pressure, kidney failure, coma.

Vitamin E

Description

Vitamin E is a pale yellow, oily, fat soluble. Includes seven tocopherals – alpha, beta, delta, epsilon, eta, gamma, zeta. Alpha tocopheral is the most effective nutritionally.

What It Does

Vitamin E is an antioxidant, preventing substances, such as Vitamin A, from immediate, uncontrolled oxidation. Increases immunity. Anticancer. Protects nerves. Anticonvulsant. Helps oxygenate blood, dilate blood vessels, and prevent blood clots. Beneficial to heart and circulatory system and to cell metabolism and repair. Used to promote fertility and prevent abortion. Also helps maintain the voluntary nervous system and involuntary muscles. As antioxidant, slows cell oxidation and aging process. Intake of fish oils increases need for Vitamin E.

Food Sources

Cold-pressed vegetable oils (corn, soy safflower, wheat germ oil), soy beans, whole wheat flour, eggs, milk, liver, lamb, pork, herring, mackerel, almonds, peanuts, apples, oranges, and *raw* vegetables including asparagus, carrots, celery, swiss chard, lettuce, kale, turnip greens, tomato, cucumber, peas, spinach.

Deficiency Effects

Abnormal fat deposits, red blood cell rupture, muscle weakness, abnormal eye movement and restricted vision, loss of muscle and reflexes, male sterility, miscarriages, premature birth. Contributes to heart and artery disease.

RDA/AI: 12 – 15 IU/15 mg.   Supplement: 30 – 200 IU/1000 mg.

Toxicity: Research continuing. May be toxic in high doses over 600 IU. May elevate blood pressure and thin blood excessively if taken with blood thinning medicines such as aspirin.

Vitamin K

Description	What It Does	Food Sources	Deficiency Effects
Vitamin K is a yellow, oily liquid.	Coenzyme of producing proteins for blood clotting and bone metabolism. Helps blood clotting by increasing prothrombin. Manufactured in intestines by bacteria. Yogurt and acidophilus milk assist this process. Synthetic Vitamin K can be harmful.	Spinach, cabbage, cauliflower, brussels sprouts, rice, bran, egg yolk, yogurt, fish liver oil, leafy green vegetables, blackstrap molasses, plant oils.	Slow blood clotting, hemorrhages, miscarriages, nosebleeds. Longterm antibiotics deplete intestinal flora effecting Vitamin K synthesis.

RDA/AI: 65 – 120 mcg.   Supplement: 50 – 100 mcg.

Toxicity: Natural Vitamin K nontoxic. Synthetic Vitamin K can damage red blood cells and brain.

Bioflavonoids

Description	What It Does	Food Sources	Deficiency Effects
Companions to Vitamin C. Antioxidants. Bioflavonoids are water soluble. There are over 500 including rutin, citrin, hesperidin, flavones, and flavonals. The vivid colors in fruits and vegetables are the bioflavonoids in the pulp and skin.	Work with Vitamin C to maintain exterior cell membranes, collagen, and capillaries and to help protect against infection and free radicals.	Fruits such as grapes, plums, blackberries, cherries, lemons, grapefruit, oranges, rosehips, buckwheat, paprika. Occurs with Vitamin C foods.	Vulnerability to bleeding, bruising, and infection.

RDA: None   Toxicity: None

MINERALS

Calcium

RDA /AI/Supplements	What It Does	Food Sources	Deficiency Effects
RDA/AI: 1000 - 1200 mg. Supplement: up to 2500 mg. Toxicity: Kidney stones. With Vitamin D, calcification of bones.	More calcium in body than any other mineral. Works with phosphorous to maintain bones and teeth. Promotes nerve transmission, muscle growth, muscle contraction, blood clotting. Helps regulate heartbeat.	Milk and milk products, green leafy vegetables, broccoli, fish, shellfish, meats, poultry, beans, fruits.	Causes bone malformation, brittle porous bones and teeth, irritability, muscle cramps, sleeplessness, depression, headaches, dementia, abnormal heartbeat.

Phosphorous

RDA/AI/Supplement	What It Does	Food Sources	Deficiency Effects
RDA/AI: 700-1000 mg Supplement: up to 4000 mg. Needs to equal calcium intake. Toxicity: Interferes with calcium absorption.	Present in every cell of the body. Works with calcium for strong bones and teeth. Helps regulate heartbeat, aids nerve transmission. Important to every metabolic process.	Protein foods such as meat, fish, eggs, poultry. Milk, yogurt, ice cream. Whole grains, beans, seeds, and nuts.	Poor bones and teeth, rickets, weight loss or gain, irregular breathing, arthritis.

Magnesium

RDA/AI/Supplement

RDA/AI: 320 – 420 mg.

Supplement: up to 500 mg. Toxicity: Excessive causes diarrhea.

Needs to equal one-half calcium intake.

What It Does

Cofactor for activating metabolic enzymes inside cells. Needed for over 300 biochemical reactions. Regulates calcium in nerves and muscle function. Helps regulate blood sugar levels. Helps maintain nervous system, nerves, heart and circulatory system.

Food Sources

Green leafy vegetables, seafood, meat, poultry, figs, seeds, nuts, corn, soybeans, yogurt, raw wheat germ, raw bran flakes, whole grains, unpolished grains, black-eye peas, potatoes, blackstrap molasses, raw fruits and berries, avocado.

Deficiency Effects

Extreme irritability, nervousness, mental disturbance, confusion, fast heartbeat, low blood pressure, muscle twitch, tremors.

Potassium

RDA/AI/Supplement

RDA/AI: 2500 – 4700 mg.

Supplement: to 4700 mg.

Must balance sodium.

Toxicity: Excess can be dangerous with kidney disease, diabetes, cardiovascular drugs.

What It Does

Maintains fluid volume inside and outside of cells. Helps regulate blood pressure in response to too much salt. Helps maintain function of nervous system, digestive system, heartbeat, muscle contractions, water balance in tissue. Helps nourish skin.

Food Sources

Lean meats, dairy, vegetables, whole grains, beans, soybeans, potatoes, tomatoes, apricots, bananas, avocado, almonds

Deficiency Effects

Slow irregular heartbeat, weakness, slow reflex, flaccid muscles, dry skin, insomnia.

Sodium

RDA/AI/Supplement	What It Does	Food Sources	Deficiency Effects
RDA/AI: 1200 – 1500 mg. Supplement: to 2300 mg. Toxicity: Body swelling, hypertension, increased risk of cardiovascular disease and stroke.	This is sodium part of sodium chloride and makes up 40% of salt by weight. Works with potassium to maintain water balance in tissue and cells. Works with chlorine to produce hydrochloric acid for stomach, helps clean carbon dioxide from body	All foods, salt, seafood, carrots, meat, poultry. (Also baking powder, baking soda.)	Uncommon. Muscle shrinkage, intestinal gas, nausea, loss of appetite.

Chloride

RDA/AI/Supplement	What It Does	Food Sources	Deficiency Effects
RDA/AI: 2300 mg. Supplement: to 3600 mg. Toxicity: Hypertension.	This is the chloride part of sodium chloride and makes up 60% of salt by weight. Helps regulate acid balance in blood. Works with sodium to maintain pressure of fluids on each side of cell wall, stimulates production of hydrochloric acid for stomach, helps liver in filtering toxicity from blood, helps maintain joints and tendons	Table salt, seaweed, seafood, rye flour, ripe olives, meats.	Digestion difficulty, poor muscle contraction. Loss of salt and fluids in perspiration in hot weather causes fatigue and heat stroke.

Iodine

RDA/AI/Supplement	What It Does	Food Sources	Deficiency Effects
RDA/AI: 150 mcg. Supplement: 1100 mcg. Toxicity: Excessive synthetic toxic. Elevated thyroid and hormone concentration.	Necessary for proper functioning of the thyroid glands in producing thyroxine, which regulates body speed and metabolism. Stimulates synthesis of cholesterol and metabolism of foods.	Ocean plant and animal foods. Iodized table salt, fish. shellfish.	Goiter or enlarged thyroid gland. Decreased stamina and vitality. Obesity, slow metabolism, slow mental processes, rapid pulse, nervousness, irritability, dry hair, hardening of arteries.

Iron

RDA/AI/Supplement	What It Does	Food Sources	Deficiency Effects
RDA/AI: 8 - 18 mg. Supplement: up to 45 mg. Toxicity: Gastrointestinal disturbance. Toxic with excessive amounts.	Forms hemoglobin in red blood cells that transports oxygen to all body cells. Component of various enzymes. Helps metabolize protein. Works with copper and calcium.	Liver, meats, poultry, oysters and seafood, eggs, molasses, spinach and other vegetables, nuts and seeds, fruits and berries, wheat bran, whole grains.	Anemia or reduced hemoglobin and oxygen to body. Fatigue, breathing difficulty.

Copper

RDA/AI/Supplement	What It Does	Food Sources	Deficiency Effects
RDA/AI: 900 mcg. Supplement: up to 10,000 mcg. Toxicity: Possible liver damage. Toxicity rare as excess is excreted.	Component of enzymes in iron metabolism helping form red blood cells. Trace mineral found in all body tissues. Helps form muscle fiber, bones, and RNA or ribonucleic acid.	Liver and organ meats, meat, poultry, seafood, eggs and dairy, fruits and berries, vegetables, beans, nuts, whole grains, cocoa, beer, tea.	Related to anemia, weakness, breathing difficulty, skin lesions.

Manganese

RDA/AI/Supplement	What It Does	Food Sources	Deficiency Effects
RDA/AI: 1.8 – 2.3 mg. Supplement: 11 mg. Toxicity: Possible with supplements, and in ample supply in drinking water along with intake of lots of vegetables. Neurotoxicity. Decrease in iron.	Trace mineral. Helps in formation of bone. Activates enzymes to metabolize B and C vitamins, carbohydrates, fatty acids, cholesterol. Aids sex hormone and breast milk production. Helps maintain brain and nervous system.	Eggs, seafood, poultry, whole grains, rice, raw fruits and vegetables, pineapple, bananas, berries, asparagus, parsley, avocado. Filberts, almonds, coconut, coffee, tea, wine, drinking water.	Glucose intolerance, lessened muscular coordination, dizziness, ear noises, hearing loss.

Selenium

RDA/AI/Supplement	What It Does	Food Sources	Deficiency Effects
RDA/AI: 55 - 70 mcg. Supplement: to 400 mcg. Toxicity: Natural, none. Synthetic, hair and nail brittleness and loss.	Trace mineral. Antioxidant regulation. Helps regulate thyroid hormone action and oxidation of Vitamin C. Maintains tissue elasticity. Antioxidant that works with Vitamin E. Detoxifier. Helps maintain fertility and normal body growth. Anticancer. Cardiovascular benefits. May be anti-aging. Amount available in foods dependent on soil.	Whole grains, wheat germ, enriched brewers yeast, eggs, milk, organ meats, seafood, molasses, cod, sole, lobster, oysters, oranges, peaches, pineapples, figs, cabbage, broccoli, carrots, corn, iceberg lettuce, mushrooms, onions, garlic, radish, tomatoes, beer, coffee, tea.	Premature aging. Growth defects. Decreased immunity. Mental retardation. Nerve disorders. Infertility.

Zinc

RDA/AI/Supplement	What It Does	Food Sources	Deficiency Effects
RDA/AI: 9 - 11 mg. Supplement: to 40 mg. Toxicity: Iron and copper loss. More Vitamin A needed.	Trace mineral throughout body. Component of many digestive enzymes, proteins, and body fluids including insulin and male-reproductive fluids. Essential to cell metabolism. Helps regulate genes. Present in white blood cells. Helps to heal wounds.	Wheat bran, whole wheat, red meats, liver, eggs, oysters, milk, poultry, raw fruits, spinach, squash, mushrooms, fortified cereals, coffee, tea, beer, dry wine.	Fatigue, slow healing of wounds, sterility, dwarfism, decreased resistance to infections.

Cobalt

RDA/AI/Supplement	What It Does	Food Sources	Deficiency Effects
RDA/AI: None Toxicity: Enlarged thyroid gland.	Part of Vitamin B12 cyanocobalamin. Helps maintain red blood cells and catalyze enzymes.	Meats, liver, poultry, clams, oysters, milk. Seaweed.	Pernicious anemia. Slow growth.

Molybdenum

RDA/AI/Supplement	What It Does	Food Sources	Deficiency Effects
RDA/AI: 45 mcg. Supplement: up to 2000 mcg. Toxicity: Copper deficiency. Reproductive effect	Helps release iron from liver storage. Helps in fat oxidation. Cofactor for enzymes in amino acid metabolism.	Whole grains, dark green leafy vegetables.	No known effects. Could help prevent and treat anemia.

Chromium

RDA/AI/Supplement	What It Does	Food Sources	Deficiency Effects
RDA/AI: 25 – 35 mcg. Supplement: 50 – 200 mcg. Toxicity: None known.	Helps maintain normal blood glucose levels. Helps activate enzymes in the metabolism of glucose, fatty acids, and cholesterol. Carries protein in the blood.	Whole grains, corn oil, meats, poultry, clams, fish, brewers yeast, beer.	Insulin dysfunction and glucose intolerance.

Fluoride

RDA/AI/Supplement	What It Does	Food Sources	Deficiency Effects
RDA/AI: 3 – 4.0 mg. Supplement: 10 mg. Toxicity: Enamel and skeletal fluorosis.	Trace mineral in tissues and primarily in bones and teeth. Facilitates calcium absorption and reduces mouth acid produced to digest carbohydrates, thereby strengthening bones and teeth. Excess is toxic, inhibiting enzymes and irritating brain tissue. Natural form is calcium fluoride. Synthetic form added to drinking water is sodium fluoride	Drinking water and seafood. Some plants, depending on soil	Tooth decay.

Vanadium

RDA/AI/Supplement	What It Does	Food Sources	Deficiency Effects
RDA: None. Toxicity: Renal lesions observed in animals.	Biological function undetermined. Trace mineral helping to regulate circulatory system. Inhibits formation of cholesterol in central nervous system and blood vessels.	Fish and seafood.	No effects known.

Boron

RDA/AI/Supplement	What It Does	Food Sources	Deficiency Effects
RDA/AI: None Supplement: 20 mg. Toxicity: Reproductive and developmental effects in animals.	No clear biological function in humans. Trace mineral may facilitate calcium absorption. May help prevent osteoporosis.	Fruit juice, potatoes, beans, milk, avocado, peanuts.	Uncommon.

Nickel

RDA/AI/Supplement	What It Does	Food Sources	Deficiency Effects
RDA/AI: None Supplement: 1 mg. Toxicity: Kidney dysfunctionals susceptible. Decreased body weight gain in animals.	Exact role unknown. Cofactor in metalloenzymes. Trace mineral found in DNA and RNA. Activates enzymes in liver, facilitates iron absorption.	Seafood, cabbage, oats, nuts, beans, seeds, cereals, sweeteners, chocolate candy, chocolate milk powder.	Effects liver function, iron metabolism, reproduction.

Recommended Daily Allowances (RDA) & Adequate Intakes (AI) for Nutrients^
Average Adult

g = gram   mg = milligram   mcg = microgram   IU = International Unitt

RE = retinol equivalent   RAE = retinol activity equivalent   Supplements: 1 RE = 1 RAE

PUF = polyunsaturated fat   LDL = low density lipoprotein (cholesterol)   HDL = high density lipoprotein

	Unit	Amount RDA/AI	Upper Levels ^ (UL)	Therapeutic Levels^^	Toxicity of Supplements (Large Amounts)
Calories	Calories	1500-2600	Maintain for weight		Excess food creates body fat
Protein	g	45-65	10 - 35% calories		May cause fluid imbalance
Carbohydrate	g	300	45 - 65% of calories		Excess creates body fat
Fat	g	60	20 - 35% calories		Excess creates body fat
Saturated Fat	g	20	Maintain low levels		Excess body fat
Polyunsaturated Fat (PUF)	g	40	Balance Omega 6 & 3		Excess Omega 6 increases LDL
Cholesterol	mg	300	Maintain low levels		Increase blood cholesterol levels
Vitamins					
Vitamin A	RE/RAE	700-900	3000		Preformed only: liver toxicity
	IU	5000	15,000	5000-10,000	Already formed toxic to pregnant
B1-Thiamine	mg	1.1 - 1.2	None	1.5 - 10	None known
B2-Riboflavin	mg	1.1 - 1.3	None	20 - 100	None known
B3-Niacin	mg	14 - 16	35	20 - 100	Over 100 mg. Skin flushes
(1200 mg *nicotinic acid*, one form of B3, for cholesterol reduction)					
B5-Pantothenic Acid*	mg	5	None	10 - 100	None known
B6-Pyridoxine	mg	1.3 - 1.7	100	50	2g+ daily toxic - no megadoses
B12-Cobalamin	mcg	2.4	None	5 to 50	None known up to 450 mg
Biotin*	mcg	30	None	100 - 300	None known
Folate/Folic Acid* **	mcg	400	1000	400 - 1000	Toxic if B12 deficient
Inositol*	mg	500-1000	prevalent in body		None known
Choline*	mg	550	3500	1000	Prolonged - B6 deficiency; liver toxicity
PABA*	mg	No RDA		30 - 100	Toxic - no high doses
Vitamin C	mg	75 - 90	2000	250-1000 2xday	Megadoses stopped - scurvy symptoms
Bioflavonoids				No RDA	
Vitamin D	IU	400	400	400 - 1000	Excrete calcium
Vitamin E	mg	15	1000		Excessive -possible hemorrhage vulnerability
	IU	30		200 - 400	600+ inhibits Vit.A, Omega 3
Vitamin K*	mcg	90 - 120	None	50 - 100	Synthetic: toxic buildup--anemia
*Synthesized by body					
Minerals					
Calcium	mg	1000-1200	2500	1000 - 1200	w/Vit D - calcification of bones
Copper	mcg	900	10,000	None	Rare - excess excreted. Liver damage.
Iron	mg	8 to 18	45	None	Toxic w/prolonged high amts
Iodine	mcg	150	1100	None	None natural/synthetic toxic
Magnesium	mg	320 - 420	350		
Magnesium needs to be 1/2 calcium			(1/2		Can be toxic in large amounts

amount				calcium)500	
Manganese	mg	1.8 - 2.3	11	None	Very high amts. neurotoxicity, less iron.
Phosphorous	mg	700	4000		Interferes with calcium absorption

Phosphorous intake should equal calcium intake.

Potassium	mg	4700	None	None	Must balance sodium
Sodium (40% of salt)	mg	1200-1500	2300	None	Swelling/hypertension-14,000-28,000mg
Chloride (60% of salt)	mg	2300	3600	None	Hypertension with excess
Selenium	mcg	55 - 70	400	50 - 200	Toxic. No more than 200 mcg. day
Zinc	mg	9 to 11	40	40	Iron & copper loss. +Vit A needed
Cobalt	mcg	No RDA		None	Enlarged thyroid gland
Chromium	mcg	25 - 35	None	50 - 200	None known.
Molybdenum	mcg	45	2000		Copper deficiency. Reproductive effects.

EAA - Essential Amino Acids

Isoleucine	mg	846	None listed
Leucine	mg	1128	None listed
Lysine	mg	875	None listed
Methionine	mg	705	None listed
Phenylalanine	mg	1128	None listed
Threonine	mg	564	None listed
Tryptophan	mg	211	None listed
Valine	mg	987	None listed
Histidine	mg	No RDA*	None listed

(Histidine (recently added for adults)

The amounts are intended as current guidelines in avoiding excess supplementation. Amounts and safe levels in supplements change as research continues.

Natural food nutrients are all safe.

^RDA & AI amounts are a compilation of those established by the US Food and Drug Administration and the National Academy of Sciences.

^Upper Levels (UL) maximum daily safe intake recommended by government.

^^ Therapeutic levels: Nutritionist safe levels.

None: No information available or no levels set.

*Manufactured in body.

**Folate is the natural occurring B vitamin in foods. Folic acid is the synthetic form in supplements and fortified foods.

KA

NUTRITION POWER

Nutrients: Liver, Brewers Yeast, Yogurt, Cottage Cheese, Wheat Germ, Wheat Germ Oil, Enriched White Flour & Bread

Liv=Liver   BY=Brewers Yeast   LFYo=Lowfat Yogurt   NFYo=Nonfat Yogurt
CC=Cottage Cheese   WG-Wheat Germ   WGO=Wheat Germ Oil
EF= Enriched Flour   EWB=Enriched White Bread   Sl=Slice   na=not available
g=grams   mg=milligrams   mcg=micrograms   IU=International Units   T=Tablespoon

Nutrient	Unit	Liv 3.5 oz	BY^ 1 T	LFYo 8 oz	NFYo 8 oz	CC1% 8 oz	WG 1 T	WGO 1 T	EF 1 T	EWB 1 Sl
Calories	Cal	190	35	143	98	162	27	120	31	67
Protein	g	29	8	12	9	28	2	0	1	2
Carbohydrates	g	5	3	16	17	6	4	0	6	12
Total Fat	g	5.3	0.1	3.5	trace	2.3	1	14	0.14	1
Saturated Fat	g	1.7		2.27	0.26	1.46	0.1	2.6	0.02	0.1
Monounsat.Fat	g	0.65		0.97	0.1	0.66	0.1	2.1	0.01	0.2
Polyunsat.Fat	g	0.64		0.1	0.01	0.07	0.4	8.4	0.06	0.5
Cholesterol	mg	396	0	13.6	5	9	0	0	0	trace

Vitamins

Nutrient	Unit	Liv 3.5 oz	BY^ 1 T	LFYo 8 oz	NFYo 8 oz	CC1% 8 oz	WG 1 T	WGO 1 T	EF 1 T	EWB 1 Sl
Vitamin A	IU	31714	trace	116	0	93	0	0	0.17	0
B1-Thiamine	mg	0.19	1.4	0.1	0.08	0.05	0.14	0	0.07	0.12
B2-Riboflavin	mg	3.43	0.7	0.49	0.37	0.37	0.04	0	0.04	0.09
B3-Niacin	mg	17.5	5.3	0.26	0.2	0.29	0.49	0	0.65	1
B5-Pantothenic*	mg	7.11	0.4	1.34	1.3	0.49	0.16	0	0.04	0.1
B6-Pyridoxine	mg	1.02	0.6	0.11	0.08	0.15	0.09	0	0.003	0.07
B12-Cobalomin	mcg	70.6	0	1.27	0.98	1.42	0	0	0	trace
Folic Acid*	mcg	0	240	0	0	0	0	0	12.84	8
Folate**	mcg	253	na	25	18		20.2	0	15.7	0.009
Biotin*	mcg	na	16	na	na	na	na	0	na	0.2
Vitamin C	mg	1.9	trace	1.8	2	0	0	0	0	0
Vitamin E	mg	0.51		0.07	0	0.02	0.94	20.3	0.03	0.23
Vitamin K*	mcg	3.3		0.5	0	0.23	0	3.4	0.03	0

Minerals

Nutrient	Unit	Liv 3.5 oz	BY^ 1 T	LFYo 8 oz	NFYo 8 oz	CC1% 8 oz	WG 1 T	WGO 1 T	EF 1 T	EWB 1 Sl
Calcium	mg	6	59	415	415	138	2.8	0	1.28	27
Phosphorous	mg	497	234	327	327	303	61	0	8.3	26
Magnesium	mg	21	33	38.6	38.6	11.3	17	0	2.1	5
Iron	mg	6.54	1.5	0.18	0.18	0.32	0.45	0	0.38	0.8
Copper	mg	14.3	0.5	0.03	0.08	0.06	0.06	0	0.02	0.03
Manganese	mg	0.36	0.13	0.009	na	0.007	0.1	0	0.07	0.07
Potassium	mg	352	222	531	326	194	64	0	8.6	30
Sodium	mg	79	60	159	133	918	0.9	0	0.17	135
Selenium	mcg	36.1	na	7.5	7	20.3	6	0	3.4	0.44
Zinc	mg	5.3	1.2	2.02	2	0.86	0.9	0	0.07	0.2

| EAAs*** | | | | | | | | | |
Nutrient	Unit	Liv 3.5 oz	BY^ 1 T	LFYo 8 oz	NFYo 8 oz	CC1% 8 oz	WG 1 T	WGO 1 T	EF 1 T	EWB 1 Sl
Tryptophan	mg	368	96	68	68	312	23	0	12	24
Threonine	mg	1215	400	490	490	1243	70	0	27	62
Isoleucine	mg	1352	400	649	649	1645	61	0	38	96
Leucine	mg	2670	694	1201	1201	2879	113	0	71	159
Lysine	mg	2247	592	1069	1069	2265	106	0	20	60
Methionine	mg	759	144	352	352	843	33	0	18	29
Phenylalanine	mg	1515	368	649	649	1510	67	0	51	108
Valine	mg	1761	480	985	985	1733	86	0	43	2

The table illustrates the concentrated nutritional power of liver, brewers yeast, yogurt, cottage
 cheese, wheat germ, and wheat germ oil (Vitamin E) compared to white flour and bread.
  Also shows how nutrients are removed during refining and why whole grains are needed.
  Many nutrients in manufactured products are from the milk products used.

Comparisons show how this diet supplies nutrition and metabolism power
 while reducing the constant need for refined white flour and shelf bread.

Nutrients vary among brands and products.

^Brewers yeast nutrients for 1 heaping tablespoon. B12 is not in yeast but is sometimes added.
Brewers yeast has 17 vitamins, 14 minerals, and 16 amino acids. It also provides RNA,
ribonucleic acid, the substance that gives cell direction or informs the cell what to do.
Brewers yeast also rich in trivalent chromium, a trace mineral that helps insulin action.

*Also manufactured in the body. Yogurt provides healthy bacteria to assist this process.
 Yogurt provides B vitamins so important to metabolic efficiency.
 Biotin is produced by body so is often not listed in nutrition charts for foods.

**Folate is the naturally occurring B vitamin. Folic Acid is the synthetic form in supplements
 and as addition to foods. The term "folate" is from the latin word "folium" for leaf.
 Folic acid is added by manufacturers to enriched flours and cereals.

***Essential Amino Acids: The proteins needed by the body from dietary sources. Histadine has
 also been recently added to the list of EAAs for adults.

Liver is a powerhouse of nutrition and is always included in sources for vitamins and minerals.
 This also illustrates the tremendous role of the liver in preparing foods for the body.

Source:
National Institutes of Health. Office of Dietary Supplements. Fact Sheets.
USDA Nutrient Data Laboratory. Food Composition. See Sources.

KA

Sources

Gebhart, Susan E. and Robin G. Thomas. *Nutritive Value of Foods*. Rev. Ed. Oct. 2002. Home and Garden Bulletin Number 72. U.S. Department of Agriculture. Agricultural Research Service. Washington, D.C.: GPO, 2002.

Hendler, Sheldon Saul, M.D., Ph.D. *The Doctors' Vitamin and Mineral Encyclopedia*. New York: Simon and Schuster, 1990.

Kirschman, Gayla J., Nutrition Search, Inc., John D. Kirschmann, Director. *Nutrition Almanac*. 4th Edition. New York: McGraw-Hill, 1996.

Kirschman, John D., Director, Nutrition Search, Inc. *Nutrition Almanac*. Rev. Ed. New York: McGraw-Hill, 1979.

National Institutes of Health. NIH Clinical Center. Office of Dietary Supplements. *Fact Sheets* http://ods.od.nih.gov/factsheets/ (2006)

Stein, Jess, Ed., *The Random House Dictionary of the English Language*. New York: Random House, 1973.

U.S Department of Agriculture. USDA Nutrient Data Laboratory. *Food Composition*. http://www.nal.usda.gov/fnic (Dec., 2003)

U.S. Department of Agriculture, Agricultural Research Service. 2005. USDA National Nutrient Database for Standard Reference, Release 18. Nutrient Data Laboratory http://www.nal.usda.gov/fnic/foodcomp/search/index.html